COMPLETE GUIDE TO UNDERSTANDING GASTRIC BYPASS SURGERY

Everything You Need To Know About Procedure, Recovery, Risks, Success Factors For Weight Loss And Improved Health

KLEIN HOYLE

Disclaimer

The content in this book is based on the author's expertise and comprehension of the topic. The author has no affiliation or link with any corporation, business, or person. This book is meant to give general information and educational material only, and it should not be interpreted as professional medical advice. Always seek the advice of a skilled healthcare expert if you have any queries about medical issues or treatments. The author and publisher expressly disclaim any responsibility resulting directly or indirectly from the use or use of the information included in this book.

Table of Contents

CHAPTER 1 13

Introduction To Gastric Bypass Surgery 13

What Is Gastric Bypass Surgery? 13

Why Is It Performed? 14

Who Is A Candidate? 14

Overview Of The Procedure 15

CHAPTER 2 17

Preparing For Surgery 17

Initial Consultation With A Surgeon...............17

Medical Evaluations And Tests 18

Dietary And Lifestyle Changes Before Surgery ..19

1. Pre-operative diet: 19

2. Lifestyle adjustments: 20

3. Vitamin and mineral supplementation:.......20

Mental Preparedness And Support..................21

CHAPTER 3 23

Understanding The Procedure 23

Types Of Gastric Bypass Surgery....................23

1. Roux-en-Y Gastric Bypass (RYGB):..........23

2. Biliopancreatic Diversion with Duodenal Switch (BPD/DS): 24

How The Surgery Is Performed# 24

   1. Anesthesia: 24

   2. Incisions: 24

   4. Rerouting the Intestines: 25

   5. Closure: 25

Risks And Benefits 25

Expected Outcomes 26

   1. Weight Loss: 26

   2. Resolution of Health Issues: 26

   3. Improved Quality of Life: 27

CHAPTER 4 29

Recovery Process 29

The Hospital Stay After Surgery 29

Pain Management 30

Diet Progression After Surgery 30

Return To Normal Activities 31

CHAPTER 5 33

Manage Diet And Nutrition 33

Modified Eating Habits Following Surgery 33

Nutritional Requirements.............................34

Vitamins And Supplements........................35

Dealing With Food Intolerances 36

CHAPTER 6 37

Long-Term Lifestyle Changes 37

Importance Of Exercise 37

Psychological Adjustments 38

Support Groups And Resources 40

Preventing Weight Gain 41

CHAPTER 7 43

Dealing With Complications 43

Potential Complications After Surgery 43

Signs To Watch For...................................46

1. Prolonged Pain: 46

3. Abnormal Bleeding: 46

4. Difficulty Breathing: 46

5. Nausea and Vomiting: 47

6. Changes in Bowel Habits:....................47

7. Nutritional deficit Symptoms:................47

When To Seek Medical Help?........................47

Strategies For Managing Complications..........49

1. Infection Control:.................................49

2. Mobility and Blood Clot Prevention:.........49

3. Nutritional Supplementation: 50

5. Regular Follow-Up and Monitoring: 50

CHAPTER 8 53

Life Following Gastric Bypass Surgery 53

Achieving And Sustaining Weight Reduction
Objectives 53

Body Image And Self-Esteem 56

Impact On Relationships................................58

Follow-Up Visits And Monitoring...................61

CHAPTER 9 65

Addressing Common Concerns......................65

Dealing With Loose Skin 65

Hair Loss Following Surgery.........................67

Changes In Taste And Appetite 68

Pregnancy Following Gastric Bypass..............70

CHAPTER 10 73

Beyond Surgery: Leading A Healthy Lifestyle....73

Implementing Healthy Habits........................73

Mindful Eating Practices...............................74

Setting Realistic Goals 75

Embracing A New Lifestyle 76

Conclusion 78

THE END 82

ABOUT THIS BOOK

The "Complete Guide to Understanding Gastric Bypass Surgery" is an invaluable reference for anybody considering or having this revolutionary treatment. From explaining the complexities of gastric bypass surgery to helping readers through the healing process and beyond, this thorough book covers every aspect of the trip with clarity and skill.

Chapter 1 introduces readers to the principles of gastric bypass surgery, including its goal, candidacy criteria, and a summary of the process itself. This fundamental information builds the foundations for educated decision-making and sets the tone for the ensuing chapters' study.

Chapter 2 focuses on the preliminary phase, stressing the significance of complete medical exams, dietary changes, and mental readiness. Patients may improve their surgery results and recover more quickly if they address these critical issues ahead of time.

Chapter 3 provides a thorough explanation of the surgical process, including the many kinds of gastric bypass procedures, related risks and advantages, and reasonable expectations for post-operative results. This educated viewpoint allows people to approach surgery with confidence and reasonable expectations.

Following surgery, Chapter 4 walks readers through the healing process, from hospitalization to pain management and progressive dietary changes. By navigating these early phases with correct counsel and care, patients may set the groundwork for long-term success.

Chapter 5 focuses on maintaining optimum nutrition and managing dietary changes, including adjusted eating habits, nutritional needs, and ways for dealing with food intolerances. Individuals may maintain their health and well-being after surgery by emphasizing dietary requirements.

Chapter 6 goes into the essential issue of long-term lifestyle changes, highlighting the value of exercise, psychological adjustment, and continuous support networks. Patients who take a holistic approach to health may reduce their chances of regaining weight and have a more happy, balanced life.

In Chapter 7, the book discusses potential consequences and provides readers with the information they need to spot warning signals and seek medical attention as soon as possible. This resource improves patient safety and confidence by equipping people to deal with anticipated difficulties ahead of time.

Chapter 8 looks at life following gastric bypass surgery, including weight reduction maintenance, body image issues, and the influence on relationships. Individuals may flourish after surgery by creating a supportive atmosphere and permitting regular monitoring.

Chapter 9 addresses frequent problems, such as loose skin and taste alterations, to ensure that readers are well-prepared for the complexities of post-operative living. By providing practical answers and comfort, the book reduces anxiety and creates a feeling of empowerment.

Finally, Chapter 10 expands beyond surgery to include the wider notion of living a healthy life, emphasizing mindful nutrition, practical goal-setting, and cultivating a sustainable lifestyle. This last chapter instills a feeling of strength and self-awareness in readers, inspiring them to embrace their newfound energy with confidence and excitement.

CHAPTER 1

Introduction To Gastric Bypass Surgery

What Is Gastric Bypass Surgery?

Gastric bypass surgery, also known as Roux-en-Y gastric bypass, is a weight-loss procedure that includes lowering the size of the stomach and rerouting the digestive tract. The technique tries to assist very obese people lose weight by restricting their food intake and lowering nutrient absorption.

Gastric bypass surgery involves the surgeon creating a tiny pouch at the top of the stomach and connecting it straight to the small intestine. This limits the quantity of food that can be ingested while bypassing a section of the stomach and the first part of the small intestine, where the majority of calories and nutrients are absorbed.

Why Is It Performed?

Gastric bypass surgery is often done on people who are severely obese and have failed to reduce weight with diet and exercise alone. Obesity causes severe health hazards, including type 2 diabetes, high blood pressure, sleep apnea, and heart disease.

The operation is not a fast cure for weight reduction, but rather a tool to assist patients in making lifestyle changes that lead to long-term weight loss and increased health. It may also assist in treating or curing obesity-related diseases including diabetes and high cholesterol.

Who Is A Candidate?

Gastric bypass surgery is often reserved for those with a body mass index (BMI) of 40 or higher, or those with a BMI of 35 or higher who have obesity-related health issues. Candidates should also have tried alternative weight-loss strategies without success and be willing to make lifestyle adjustments following surgery.

Candidates for gastric bypass surgery are often evaluated thoroughly by a multidisciplinary team that includes a surgeon, dietician, psychologist, and other healthcare specialists. This examination determines if the person is physically and emotionally prepared for surgery and able to follow post-operative instructions.

Overview Of The Procedure

Gastric bypass surgery is often performed under general anesthesia and may be accomplished using minimally invasive procedures like laparoscopy, which involves creating tiny incisions in the abdomen.

During the surgery, the surgeon forms a tiny pouch at the top of the stomach using surgical staples or a band. This pouch is then attached straight to the small intestine, skipping the remainder of the stomach and the first section of the small intestine.

Gastric bypass surgery, which lowers the size of the stomach and bypasses a section of the digestive system, limits the quantity of food that can be consumed and minimizes calorie and nutritional absorption. This results in weight reduction and improves or resolves obesity-related health problems.

Patients are often admitted to the hospital for a few days after surgery for monitoring and recuperation. They will need to adhere to a rigorous diet and fitness regimen, as well as taking nutritional supplements, to guarantee optimum healing and long-term success. Regular follow-up meetings with healthcare experts are also required to monitor development and handle any issues or difficulties.

CHAPTER 2

Preparing For Surgery

Initial Consultation With A Surgeon

The path to gastric bypass surgery often begins with an initial consultation with a surgeon. This is an important phase in which you will consult with a medical specialist who specializes in bariatric surgery to explore your choices and decide if you are a good candidate for the treatment. During this meeting, the surgeon will inquire about your medical history, prior weight reduction efforts, current health condition, and the reasons for choosing gastric bypass surgery.

The surgeon will also do a medical examination to check your general health and identify any underlying disorders that might compromise the procedure or its consequences. This may entail determining your weight, height, and BMI (Body Mass Index), as well as screening for diabetes, high blood pressure, or sleep apnea.

Additionally, the first meeting allows you to ask any concerns you may have regarding the procedure, its risks and advantages, the recuperation process, and what to anticipate in the long run. It is important to be upfront and honest with your surgeon during this appointment to ensure that you get the best possible treatment and obtain the desired results from the operation.

Medical Evaluations And Tests

Following the first appointment, you will be subjected to a battery of medical tests and examinations to establish your overall health and suitability for gastric bypass surgery. These assessments may involve blood tests, imaging tests like X-rays or ultrasounds, and maybe an electrocardiogram (ECG) to examine your heart function.

These tests are necessary for detecting any possible dangers or issues that may develop before or after surgery, as well as confirming that you are in good enough health to undertake the treatment. Your surgeon will go over the findings of these tests with you in detail, including any extra measures that may be required before continuing with the operation.

Dietary And Lifestyle Changes Before Surgery

You will need to make major dietary and lifestyle adjustments before having gastric bypass surgery. These improvements are critical for improving surgical results and lowering the risk of complications. Your surgeon or certified dietician will give you specific suggestions to follow, which might include:

1. **Pre-operative diet:** You may be put on a particular diet to help shrink your liver and lower the amount of fat in your belly, making the operation safer and simpler to conduct.

This diet often consists of ingesting a low-calorie, high-protein liquid diet for some time before surgery.

2. Lifestyle adjustments: In addition to food changes, you may be encouraged to stop smoking, limit alcohol use, and increase physical activity. These modifications are critical for enhancing your general health and lowering the likelihood of problems before and after surgery.

3. Vitamin and mineral supplementation: Gastric bypass surgery may impair the absorption of certain vitamins and minerals, resulting in shortages if not treated correctly. You may be given vitamin and mineral supplements to take before and after surgery to avoid deficiencies and promote overall health.

4. Psychological preparation is a vital part of preparing for gastric bypass surgery. You may be asked to undertake psychiatric examinations or therapy to determine your preparation for the surgery and to assist you in dealing with any emotional or

psychological issues that may develop during the preoperative time.

Mental Preparedness And Support

Gastric bypass surgery is a significant life shift, and it is typical to feel a variety of emotions throughout the preoperative period. Mental preparation and support are critical in helping you deal with the difficulties and uncertainties of the procedure.

Your healthcare staff may suggest individual or group therapy sessions to help you address any fears or anxiety you may have about the operation, as well as to teach you coping methods for dealing with stress and emotions.

In addition to professional help, it's crucial to seek emotional support from friends and family at this time. A solid support network may greatly improve your capacity to manage the pre-operative time and prepare mentally and emotionally for surgery.

Overall, preparing for gastric bypass surgery requires a holistic strategy that covers not just the physical components of the treatment but also its psychological and emotional implications. Working closely with your healthcare team and making the appropriate lifestyle modifications may boost your chances of success while also improving your general health and well-being.

CHAPTER 3

Understanding The Procedure

Types Of Gastric Bypass Surgery

When contemplating gastric bypass surgery, it is important to understand the many options available. The two most common kinds are Roux-en-Y gastric bypass (RYGB) and biliopancreatic diversion with duodenal switch (BPD/DS).

1. Roux-en-Y Gastric Bypass (RYGB): This is the most often performed gastric bypass operation. During RYGB, the surgeon staples the top region of the stomach to form a tiny pouch, therefore lowering its size. A piece of the small intestine is then linked to the pouch, skipping the remainder of the stomach and the top portion of the small intestine. This rerouting decreases the quantity of food you may consume and the absorption of nutrients.

2. Biliopancreatic Diversion with Duodenal Switch (BPD/DS): This is a more difficult treatment that is usually reserved for those with a higher BMI. BPD/DS entails removing a substantial section of the stomach to form a smaller pouch, comparable to RYGB. However, in BPD/DS, a considerable portion of the small intestine is skipped, significantly limiting calorie and nutrient absorption.

How The Surgery Is Performed#

Gastric bypass surgery is often done laparoscopically, which is a minimally invasive procedure that involves creating many tiny incisions in the belly. Here's a step-by-step explanation of the procedure:

1. Anesthesia: General anesthetic will be administered to keep you asleep and pain-free throughout the procedure.

2. Incisions: The surgeon will make multiple tiny incisions in your abdomen to get access to your stomach and intestines.

3. The surgeon will split the stomach using surgical staples or a stapling instrument, resulting in a tiny pouch at the top. This pouch will serve as your new stomach for holding meals.

4. **Rerouting the Intestines:** The small intestine is separated, and the bottom piece is raised and attached to the newly formed stomach pouch. This permits food to skip the remainder of the stomach and the upper section of the small intestine.

5. **Closure:** The incisions are closed with sutures or surgical staples, and the wounds are covered with sterile cloths.

Risks And Benefits

Gastric bypass, like any other operation, has dangers and advantages that should be carefully considered before going.

Infection, hemorrhage, blood clots, surgical leaks, and nutritional deficits are all potential risks. There is also a danger of problems from anesthesia.

Benefits: Gastric bypass surgery may help you lose weight and improve or resolve obesity-related health issues including type 2 diabetes, hypertension, and sleep apnea. It may also increase general well-being and self-esteem.

Expected Outcomes

The predicted effects of gastric bypass surgery vary from person to person, but often include:

1. **Weight Loss:** Most people may anticipate losing a lot of weight in the first year after surgery. Patients may often lose 60% to 80% of their extra body weight in 18 to 24 months.

2. **Resolution of Health Issues:** Following gastric bypass surgery, several obesity-related health issues, such as

type 2 diabetes, high blood pressure, and high cholesterol, generally improve or disappear entirely.

3. **Improved Quality of Life:** Patients often report increased mobility, energy, mood, and self-confidence after major weight reduction.

Understanding the many forms of gastric bypass surgery, the surgical operation itself, possible risks and advantages, and anticipated results will help you make an educated choice about whether this is the best option for you. Always talk with a certified healthcare expert about your specific situation and treatment choices.

CHAPTER 4

Recovery Process

The Hospital Stay After Surgery

The hospital stay after gastric bypass surgery normally lasts one to three days, depending on the individual's recovery progress and probable problems. After surgery, patients are carefully observed in the recovery area before being transported to a hospital room.

Throughout the hospital stay, medical professionals will manage pain, provide antibiotics to avoid infection, and constantly check vital signs. Patients cannot ingest solid food shortly after surgery, thus intravenous fluids are administered to avoid dehydration.

Patients are recommended to get exercise as soon as possible to avoid blood clots and enhance recovery. Nurses and other medical personnel will help patients move and do other activities as required.

Pain Management

Pain management is an important part of the rehabilitation process after gastric bypass surgery. Patients may feel pain, particularly in the abdomen region, for many days after the treatment. Doctors may prescribe pain relievers both in the hospital and at home throughout the healing phase.

Patients must strictly adhere to the specified drug schedule and notify their healthcare practitioner immediately if they have severe or increasing discomfort. In addition to medicine, putting cold packs at the surgery site may help minimize swelling and pain.

Diet Progression After Surgery

Diet progression is a progressive procedure that begins with clear liquids and progresses to solid meals over a few weeks. Patients are only permitted to consume clear liquids such as water, broth, and sugar-free gelatin immediately after surgery. Patients may introduce pureed and soft meals gradually as their bodies recover and acclimate to their new stomach size.

Following the advice of a certified dietician is critical during this time to promote optimum nutrition and recuperation. Patients must eat enough protein to promote recovery and avoid muscle loss. Vitamin and mineral supplements may also be prescribed to avoid nutritional deficits.

Return To Normal Activities

Returning to regular activities following gastric bypass surgery varies from person to person and is determined by the individual's healing process. Most patients may return to mild activities, such as walking, within a few days following surgery. However, excessive activity and heavy lifting should be avoided for several weeks to enable the body to fully recover.

Patients should adhere to their surgeon's suggestions for returning to work and other everyday activities. It's critical to listen to your body and prevent overexertion throughout the recuperation period. Gradually increasing exercise as tolerated may assist in avoiding difficulties and ensure a smooth recovery.

Patients who follow the specified pain management plan, adhere to the recommended diet progression, and gradually return to regular activities may help their recovery and achieve satisfactory results after gastric bypass surgery.

CHAPTER 5

Manage Diet And Nutrition

Modified Eating Habits Following Surgery

Gastric bypass surgery significantly affects how your body processes food, demanding considerable dietary changes. Initially, you'll go through many phases of dietary progression, beginning with clear liquids and progressively reintroducing solid meals. Your surgeon and nutritionist will offer precise suggestions based on your requirements, but in general, you'll begin with small, frequent meals to improve digestion and reduce pain.

Portion control becomes critical after surgery. Because your stomach is tiny, it can only contain small quantities of food at once, so you must eat slowly and chew carefully to avoid issues such as nausea or vomiting.

Adopting a balanced diet rich in lean meats, vegetables, fruits, and whole grains is critical for satisfying your nutritional requirements while also boosting weight reduction and general health.

Nutritional Requirements

Meeting your dietary requirements after gastric bypass surgery is critical for maintaining energy, promoting recovery, and avoiding shortages. Your smaller stomach restricts meal intake, so it's critical to pick nutrient-dense options. Protein takes primacy because it promotes muscle repair, immunological function, and satiety. Lean meats, fish, eggs, dairy, lentils, and protein supplements are all good sources.

Vitamins and minerals are very important for post-bypass health. While a well-balanced diet should include many vital elements, supplementation is often required to avoid shortages. Calcium, vitamin D, vitamin B12, iron, and folate are among the most important nutrients.

Regular blood tests will monitor your levels and enable you to change your supplement program as required.

Vitamins And Supplements

Because of the changed architecture and decreased food intake after surgery, many patients need lifetime supplements to maintain good health. Vitamin and mineral deficits are prevalent following gastric bypass, requiring the daily use of prescription supplements to avoid problems such as anemia, osteoporosis, and neurological diseases.

Calcium and vitamin D are essential for bone health, and they are often taken together to improve absorption. Vitamin B12 is required for nerve function and red blood cell synthesis, while iron helps to prevent anemia. Folate is important for DNA synthesis and cell proliferation. Your healthcare team will recommend the best supplement regimen for you based on your specific requirements, and you will have frequent blood tests to check your levels.

Dealing With Food Intolerances

Certain meals may become difficult to stomach after a gastric bypass because of changes in your digestive tract. Foods heavy in sugar or fat may trigger dumping syndrome, which is characterized by a fast heart rate, perspiration, nausea, and diarrhea. Carbonated drinks and fibrous foods may also cause pain or obstructions.

Identifying and avoiding troublesome foods is critical for reducing pain and improving nutrition. Keeping a food journal might help you identify triggers and make educated nutritional decisions. Experimenting with various textures and cooking techniques may enhance tolerability while collaborating closely with your healthcare team provides continuing support and assistance in successfully managing food intolerances.

CHAPTER 6

Long-Term Lifestyle Changes

Importance Of Exercise

Exercise is critical to the long-term effectiveness of gastric bypass surgery. It not only assists in weight reduction but also promotes general health and well-being. Patients recovering from surgery may find it difficult to participate in physical exercise at first owing to low energy levels and various physical restrictions. However, as they recuperate and adjust to their new lifestyle, exercise becomes more crucial.

Regular exercise helps to burn calories, increase metabolism, and develop muscle mass, all of which aid in weight reduction and maintenance. It also promotes cardiovascular health, bone strength, stress reduction, and mood enhancement. Patients are urged to begin with low-impact activities like walking, swimming, or cycling, then progressively increase the intensity and time as tolerated.

Physical exercise improves both the body and the mind. Endorphins, which are natural mood enhancers, are released during exercise, assisting patients in combating feelings of despair and anxiety that are frequent with obesity and major life changes such as surgery. As patients' strength, endurance, and general fitness levels increase, they feel a feeling of success and gain self-esteem.

Psychological Adjustments

Gastric bypass surgery not only alters the body but also necessitates considerable psychological changes. Patients may feel a variety of emotions before and during surgery, including enthusiasm, worry, irritation, and even grief. Patients must address their emotions and build coping techniques to overcome the hurdles of weight reduction and lifestyle change.

One frequent psychological adjustment after gastric bypass surgery is establishing a new connection with eating. Patients must relearn eating patterns, portion management, and mindful eating to avoid overeating or relapsing to harmful behaviors. They may also have emotional eating triggers and must develop new coping strategies to cope with stress or boredom.

Furthermore, body image difficulties may occur when people lose weight quickly and alter their physical appearance. Patients must concentrate on the positive parts of their transition and celebrate their accomplishments along the way. Seeking help from mental health specialists, support groups, or individuals who have been through similar circumstances may all give vital direction and encouragement throughout this process.

Support Groups And Resources

Support groups contribute significantly to the long-term success of gastric bypass surgery by offering patients encouragement, assistance, and a feeling of community. These organizations may include other patients, healthcare professionals, or internet forums devoted to weight reduction surgery. They provide a forum for patients to discuss their experiences, seek guidance, and provide assistance to others suffering similar issues.

In addition to support groups, there are a variety of tools available to assist patients with their post-operative journey. These might include nutritional counseling, fitness programs, culinary lessons, and instructional sessions on issues like meal planning, grocery shopping, and behavior adjustment. Healthcare practitioners may also give personalized coaching and follow-up treatment to track patients' development and address any problems that may emerge.

Patients are advised to use these tools to remain motivated, informed, and accountable on their weight reduction journey. Building a solid support network and arming oneself with the essential tools and information may considerably improve the chances of long-term success after gastric bypass surgery.

Preventing Weight Gain

While gastric bypass surgery may result in considerable weight reduction, sustaining the benefits needs consistent work and dedication. One of the most difficult issues that patients may encounter is avoiding weight regain, which may be caused by a variety of variables including lifestyle behaviors, food choices, and metabolic changes.

To avoid weight regain, patients must make long-term lifestyle adjustments and follow their post-operative instructions. This involves eating a well-balanced diet, getting regular exercise, keeping hydrated, and emphasizing self-care. To avoid overeating, patients should consume nutrient-dense meals, avoid processed or high-calorie foods, and use portion control techniques.

In addition to lifestyle changes, frequent follow-up meetings with healthcare experts are critical for tracking success, resolving issues, and making necessary adjustments. Patients may also benefit from continued assistance from dietitians, psychologists, or support groups to keep them motivated and responsible.

Patients may reduce their risk of weight return and achieve long-term success after gastric bypass surgery by being vigilant of their food and lifestyle choices, getting help when necessary, and prioritizing their health and well-being.

CHAPTER 7

Dealing With Complications

Potential Complications After Surgery

Gastric bypass surgery, like other major surgical procedures, has risks and problems. While the surgery is typically safe, it is crucial to be aware of any potential side effects that may occur during recovery and beyond.

One significant hazard is the possibility of infection at the surgical site. This may happen when germs infiltrate the incision site during or after surgery. An infection may cause redness, swelling, warmth, and discomfort around the incision site. In extreme situations, fever and pus discharge may also occur. It is critical to thoroughly monitor the surgery site for any indications of infection and report them to your doctor right away.

Another frequent risk is the formation of blood clots, commonly known as deep vein thrombosis (DVT), usually in the legs. Patients are typically less mobile after surgery, which increases the risk of blood clots developing in the deep veins of the legs. DVT symptoms might include discomfort, edema, redness, and warmth in the afflicted limb. In certain situations, a blood clot may break away and migrate to the lungs, resulting in a pulmonary embolism, a potentially fatal illness. As a result, it is critical to be aware of these symptoms and seek medical assistance immediately if they arise.

Furthermore, gastric bypass surgery may cause nutritional shortages if proper food and supplement consumption is not maintained. Because the surgery affects the digestive tract, it may reduce the body's capacity to absorb certain nutrients, including vitamin B12, iron, calcium, and folate. Without adequate supplementation, patients may have deficient symptoms such as tiredness, weakness, hair loss, and neurological issues. Nutrient levels should be monitored regularly, and prescribed supplementation requirements should be followed to avoid deficiencies and promote optimum health after surgery.

Furthermore, problems from the surgical operation itself, such as leaks or strictures, may develop in rare circumstances. A leak may form at the surgical connection site, allowing digestive juices to enter the abdominal cavity and cause infection and other significant consequences. Symptoms of a leak may include stomach discomfort, fever, fast heart rate, and trouble breathing. Similarly, strictures, or constriction of the newly formed stomach pouch or intestine, may cause blockage and difficulties in passing food. Strictures may cause nausea, vomiting, and trouble swallowing. Prompt medical care is required to treat these issues and prevent them from recurring.

Signs To Watch For

Following gastric bypass surgery, it is critical to be watchful and look for any indications or symptoms that may signal a problem. Some of the major indications to look for are:

1. **Prolonged Pain:** Any prolonged or severe pain, particularly at the surgery site or in the belly, should be checked by a healthcare specialist right once.

2. A fever may suggest an infection or some underlying issue, especially if it is accompanied by chills, sweating, or exhaustion.

3. **Abnormal Bleeding:** If you have excessive bleeding from the surgery site or elsewhere, contact your healthcare professional right once.

4. **Difficulty Breathing:** Difficulty breathing, shortness of breath, or chest discomfort may suggest a pulmonary embolism or another respiratory issue and need prompt medical intervention.

5. Nausea and Vomiting: While some nausea and vomiting are normal in the early stages of recovery, persistent or severe symptoms should be investigated by a healthcare practitioner since they may suggest a complication such as a stricture or intestinal blockage.

6. Changes in Bowel Habits: Serious changes in bowel habits, such as diarrhea, constipation, or bloody stools, should be reported to your doctor since they may suggest a gastrointestinal problem or infection.

7. Nutritional deficit Symptoms: Fatigue, weakness, hair loss, and neurological disorders are all signs of a nutritional deficit that should be treated as soon as possible with supplements and dietary changes.

When To Seek Medical Help?

If you suffer any of the aforementioned signs or symptoms, get medical attention right once. Do not ignore or dismiss any troubling symptoms, since early attention might prevent issues from developing and speed up recovery.

In general, you should seek emergency medical assistance if you feel:

• Persistent or severe stomach discomfort.

• Fever of 101°F (38.3°C) or higher.

• Difficulty breathing or chest discomfort.

• Excessive bleeding.

• Persistent vomiting or difficulty retaining fluids.

• Signs of dehydration include dark urine, dry mouth, and dizziness.

• Sudden onset of severe headache and disorientation.

If you're uncertain about any symptoms you're having, it's always a good idea to seek medical attention. Your healthcare practitioner may analyze your condition and, if required, recommend you to a specialist.

Strategies For Managing Complications

Managing difficulties following gastric bypass surgery often requires a collaborative effort among healthcare experts such as surgeons, dietitians, and other specialists. Here are some techniques for dealing with typical difficulties.

1. Infection Control: Proper wound care and cleanliness may help avoid surgical site infections. This involves keeping the incision clean and dry, according to the post-operative care recommendations given by your healthcare team, and quickly reporting any indications of infection to your physician.

2. Mobility and Blood Clot Prevention: Moving about as soon as feasible after surgery and adhering to a specified routine of leg exercises may help avoid blood clots. In addition, to lower the risk of DVT, your healthcare professional may suggest compression stockings or blood thinners.

3. Nutritional Supplementation: Following suggested supplementation recommendations and diet changes is critical for avoiding nutritional deficits. This may involve taking vitamin and mineral supplements as recommended, eating nutrient-dense meals, and getting frequent blood tests to check nutrient levels.

4. Prompt Medical Intervention for Surgical Consequences: If a surgical complication arises, such as a leak or stricture, immediate medical attention is required to manage the problem and avoid subsequent consequences. The form and severity of the problem may need further surgical operations, endoscopic techniques, or other therapies.

5. Regular Follow-Up and Monitoring: Scheduling regular follow-up sessions with your healthcare practitioner is critical for tracking your progress, resolving any concerns or issues that occur, and making any changes to your treatment plan. Your healthcare team can give direction and support throughout your rehabilitation process, ensuring the greatest possible results.

By being watchful, obtaining immediate medical help when necessary, and according to your healthcare team's recommendations, you may successfully manage difficulties after gastric bypass surgery and encourage successful recovery. Remember to speak freely with your healthcare professionals about any concerns or symptoms you are experiencing, as early action is critical to reducing the effect of problems and maximizing your long-term health and well-being.

CHAPTER 8

Life Following Gastric Bypass Surgery

Achieving And Sustaining Weight Reduction Objectives

After gastric bypass surgery, patients' major emphasis is on reaching and maintaining their weight reduction objectives. The procedure modifies the digestive system by lowering the size of the stomach and rerouting the intestines, which has a substantial impact on how the body processes food and absorbs nutrients. While the process might help you lose weight quickly, it's important to remember that long-term success takes dedication and lifestyle modifications.

Following the eating plan given by healthcare specialists is one of the first steps toward attaining weight reduction objectives after surgery. Patients begin on a liquid diet, then progress to pureed meals before returning to solid foods. Portion management is critical since the smaller stomach pouch can only store a certain quantity of food. Eating slowly and completely improves digestion and reduces pain.

Regular exercise is another important factor in weight reduction success after gastric bypass surgery. Physical exercise not only burns calories but also promotes lean muscle mass, which enhances metabolism. It's critical to begin softly and progressively increase the intensity and length of exercises as tolerated. Finding pleasant and sustainable activities will help you stick to your fitness plan.

Monitoring food consumption and making healthy choices are essential for sustaining weight reduction over time. This includes limiting portion sizes, eating nutrient-dense meals, and avoiding empty calories from sugary and processed foods. Keeping a food diary may help you monitor your eating habits and find areas for improvement. Furthermore, maintaining hydrated by drinking enough of water throughout the day is critical for general health and avoiding dehydration, particularly with a smaller stomach capacity.

Support from healthcare specialists, such as dietitians and psychologists, may be very beneficial in attaining weight reduction objectives after surgery. They may help with meal planning, behavior modification tactics, and coping skills for dealing with emotional eating or food cravings. Support groups, both in-person and online, provide encouragement and accountability as patients negotiate their weight-loss journey.

Reaching and sustaining weight reduction objectives after gastric bypass surgery needs commitment, discipline, and support. Patients may achieve long-term success and enhance their overall health and well-being by adhering to a structured diet plan, engaging in regular exercise, making good food choices, and getting help from healthcare experts and organizations.

Body Image And Self-Esteem

Gastric bypass surgery causes both physical and psychological changes. While the surgery may result in significant weight reduction and better health results, individuals often suffer mixed emotions and difficulties as a consequence of their altered look and sense of self.

One of the most noticeable side effects of gastric bypass surgery is fast weight reduction, which may result in loose skin and body shape abnormalities. Excess skin may be a tangible sign of development, but it can also be uncomfortable and make you self-conscious. Body contouring operations may be an option for some patients to remove extra skin and boost body confidence, but it is critical to talk with a plastic surgeon about the risks and advantages.

Another part of body image and self-esteem after surgery is adapting to a new identity as a "smaller" person.

Patients may experience emotions of skepticism or uneasiness as they adjust to their new bodies and navigate social situations. Individuals should concentrate on the benefits of their weight reduction journey, such as better health and mobility, rather than just on exterior appearance.

Creating a healthy body image and boosting self-esteem after gastric bypass surgery entails more than simply physical improvements. It necessitates treating underlying emotional difficulties and developing self-confidence from within. Counseling or therapy may assist individuals battling with body image problems by allowing them to examine their emotions, create coping techniques, and promote self-compassion.

Support from loved ones and friends are also important in developing a good body image and self-esteem after surgery. Encouragement and affirmation from friends and family members may increase confidence and give comfort in difficult situations. Connecting with others who have had similar experiences, whether via support groups or online forums, may also provide empathy, understanding, and solidarity.

Body image and self-esteem are complicated concerns that demand attention and care after gastric bypass surgery. While physical changes may be noticeable, patients must concentrate on their entire well-being and accept their new identities as healthier, more resilient persons. As they continue their weight reduction journey, patients may create a strong sense of self-esteem and body confidence by obtaining assistance from healthcare experts, participating in counseling or therapy, and establishing good interactions with others.

Impact On Relationships

Gastric bypass surgery impacts not just the person receiving the process, but also their relationships with family, friends, and love partners. Lifestyle changes looks, and priorities after surgery may put a strain on existing relationships, necessitating adjustment and open communication to keep them healthy.

One of the most visible effects of gastric bypass surgery on relationships is a shift in social dynamics around food and eating habits. Patients may be unable to engage in shared meals or social events based on food as they did before surgery. If friends and family members are not understanding or supportive of dietary limitations, you may feel alone or excluded.

Furthermore, changes in looks and self-confidence after surgery might affect how people interact with others and see themselves in relationships. Some patients may gain confidence and assertiveness, whilst others may feel vulnerable or insecure. As patients go through these emotional shifts, loved ones should give comfort and acceptance.

Communication is essential in managing the effects of gastric bypass surgery on relationships. Patients and loved ones should communicate honestly about their experiences, problems, and needs. This might include establishing limits around food-related activities, finding alternate ways to spend time together that do not focus on eating and addressing any issues or fears that emerge.

Support from loved ones may make a big difference in how patients adapt to life after gastric bypass surgery and handle relationship adjustments. Encouragement, empathy, and understanding may help to develop ties and provide a feeling of connection during times of change and adjustment. Both patients and loved ones must approach the post-surgery path with tolerance, compassion, and flexibility.

Gastric bypass surgery may have a significant influence on relationships, necessitating openness, understanding, and communication to sustain good bonds. Patients and their loved ones may traverse the post-surgery journey with sensitivity and support by noticing and resolving changes in social dynamics, appearance, and mental well-being, therefore enhancing their connections.

Follow-Up Visits And Monitoring

After gastric bypass surgery, follow-up checkups and monitoring are critical for long-term success and health maintenance. These consultations enable healthcare experts to evaluate progress, handle any issues or concerns, and provide patients with continuous support and assistance as they embark on their weight reduction journey.

In the initial post-operative period, follow-up consultations are usually planned regularly to evaluate healing and ensure patients are responding well to their new food and lifestyle habits. This might involve evaluating weight reduction progress, nutritional health, and any consequences including infection or vitamin deficits. Patients are also taught the necessity of following dietary rules, taking prescribed medicines, and participating in regular physical exercise.

Follow-up sessions grow less frequent over time, but they are still necessary for monitoring long-term results and treating any difficulties that occur. Healthcare experts may monitor weight reduction trends, do blood tests to measure nutritional status, and give continuous support and direction to assist patients in achieving and maintaining their weight loss goals and general health.

In addition to medical monitoring, long-term success following gastric bypass surgery requires the help of multidisciplinary healthcare teams, which include nutritionists, psychologists, and exercise physiologists. These specialists may provide personalized advice on food, exercise, behavior modification, and mental well-being, addressing the complex requirements of patients going through major lifestyle changes.

Patients are urged to actively participate in their healthcare by attending follow-up visits, following prescribed treatment regimens, and speaking for their needs and concerns.

Open communication with healthcare practitioners is critical for dealing with problems or difficulties quickly and efficiently.

In conclusion, follow-up visits and monitoring are critical components of long-term success after gastric bypass surgery. Patients who remain active in their healthcare and collaborate with multidisciplinary healthcare teams may get the support and direction they need to accomplish and maintain their weight reduction goals, as well as maximize their overall health and well-being.

CHAPTER 9

Addressing Common Concerns

Dealing With Loose Skin

Loose skin is a typical problem among patients after gastric bypass surgery. This problem originates as a result of the fast weight loss that occurs after surgery, which might prevent the skin from properly contracting to the new body size. While loose skin may be irritating and undermine one's confidence, there are numerous solutions to this problem.

One alternative is to allow your body time to adapt naturally. As you continue to lose weight and live a healthy lifestyle, your skin may gradually adjust to your new form. However, this process might take time, and natural adaptation alone does not provide good outcomes for everyone.

Another option is to integrate strength training activities into your workout regimen. Muscle building may assist in filling up slack skin and make your body seem more toned. Concentrate on workouts for regions prone to loose skin, such as the belly, arms, and thighs. Furthermore, keeping your skin moisturized and moisturizing daily might help to enhance its elasticity and look.

In certain circumstances, people may choose surgical techniques to remove extra skin. These operations, often known as body contouring or skin removal surgery, entail removing extra skin and tightening the remaining skin to achieve a smoother, more contoured look. While these operations may have spectacular outcomes, they are invasive treatments that must be carefully planned and discussed with a trained physician.

It's crucial to realize that coping with loose skin is an individual experience, and what works for one person may not work for another. It's important to be patient with your body and concentrate on total health and well-being rather than just beauty.

Hair Loss Following Surgery

Hair loss is a frequent occurrence after gastric bypass surgery, usually commencing three to six months after the procedure. Telogen effluvium is a transient condition induced by physical stress, such as fast weight loss and nutritional intake fluctuations.

While hair loss might be upsetting, it's essential to remember that it's often transient and reversible. Hair growth usually returns within six to twelve months after surgery, as your body adapts to the alterations and your weight stabilizes.

To reduce hair loss and promote healthy hair growth, emphasize good diet and hydration. Make sure you're getting enough protein, vitamins, and minerals, since deficits may worsen hair loss.

Staying hydrated and eating a well-balanced diet may also improve scalp health and encourage hair growth.

In rare circumstances, healthcare practitioners may offer biotin or iron supplements to promote hair health. However, it is critical to contact your healthcare provider before beginning any new supplements, since individual requirements may differ.

While hair loss might be alarming, it is important to consider the overall picture of increased health and well-being that comes with gastric bypass surgery. Remember that hair loss is generally transitory and will gradually improve as your body adapts to its new normal.

Changes In Taste And Appetite

Following gastric bypass surgery, many patients report changes in taste and appetite, which may have a considerable influence on their eating choices. These alterations are often related to the changed structure of the digestive system and hormonal imbalances that occur after surgery.

One frequent alteration is a decreased tolerance for certain meals, particularly those heavy in sugar, fat, or carbs. Many patients discover that they no longer like or can tolerate items they previously sought, such as sweets or oily meals. This alteration in taste preferences may be good for weight reduction and long-term health, but it may need changes in meal planning and food selection.

In addition, some patients report a reduction in appetite or sensations of fullness after consuming small quantities of food. This shift is caused by a smaller stomach and changing hormone levels, which communicate satiety to the brain. While this may help with weight reduction, it's important to make sure you're getting enough nutrients to support your general health and well-being.

To successfully manage these changes, concentrate on nutrient-dense meals that provide important vitamins, minerals, and protein. Include a mix of fruits, vegetables, lean meats, and whole grains in your meals to guarantee appropriate nutrition while accommodating variations in taste and appetite.

It's also important to listen to your body and respect its hunger and fullness signals. Eat slowly, chew deeply, and quit eating when you're content, not stuffed. Developing attentive eating habits may help you make better choices and achieve long-term success after gastric bypass surgery.

Pregnancy Following Gastric Bypass

There are numerous essential variables to consider while contemplating pregnancy after gastric bypass surgery. Pregnancy after gastric bypass is conceivable, but it must be approached with caution and an understanding of potential risks and problems.

One thing to think about is how fast weight loss and changes in nutritional status may affect fertility. Women who have had gastric bypass surgery may have better fertility owing to weight reduction and improved hormonal balance. Before trying to conceive, you must first verify that you are in excellent general health and have attained weight stability.

Pregnancy may also influence the results of weight reduction surgery. Pregnancy increases the body's stress and may impair vitamin absorption, thus affecting weight loss or nutritional status. It is important to collaborate closely with your healthcare team to assess your health and nutritional condition during pregnancy and make any required changes to your diet or medical treatment.

Furthermore, pregnancy following gastric bypass surgery may include higher risks such as nutritional deficits, gestational diabetes, and intrauterine growth limitation.

Discuss these risks with your healthcare practitioner and create a prenatal care plan that covers your specific needs and concerns.

Despite these hurdles, many women can conceive and have healthy babies after gastric bypass surgery. Pregnancy after weight reduction surgery may be a safe and gratifying experience with adequate planning, monitoring, and support from healthcare specialists.

CHAPTER 10

Beyond Surgery: Leading A Healthy Lifestyle

Implementing Healthy Habits

Following gastric bypass surgery, implementing healthy behaviors into your daily routine is critical for long-term success. These routines not only help you lose weight, but they also improve your entire health. Maintaining a healthy diet is one of the most important habits to follow. This includes eating lean meats, fruits, vegetables, and whole grains while avoiding refined sweets and processed meals. Planning meals ahead of time and having healthy snacks on hand might help you maintain better eating habits.

Regular physical exercise is another important component of a healthy lifestyle after surgery. It not only helps with weight loss but also improves cardiovascular health, mood, and energy levels.

Starting with low-impact workouts like walking or swimming and progressively increasing intensity and duration as tolerated might help you gain strength and endurance over time. Finding things that you like makes it simpler to maintain motivation and consistency.

In addition to food and exercise, proper hydration is essential for post-surgery recovery. Drinking enough of water throughout the day prevents dehydration, improves digestion, and increases satiety. It is important to drink water moderately between meals to prevent overfilling the stomach pouch and creating pain. It is also recommended to avoid sugary drinks and excessive caffeine consumption.

Mindful Eating Practices

Practicing mindful eating is an important skill for those who have had gastric bypass surgery. Mindful eating entails paying attention to hunger and fullness signs, eating carefully, and enjoying every meal. This method reduces overeating and improves better digestion. It also fosters a greater appreciation for food and promotes healthy eating habits.

Another part of mindful eating is being aware of one's emotional eating triggers. Many individuals rely on food for comfort or to deal with stress, boredom, or other emotions. Learning alternate coping techniques, such as meditation, journaling, or seeking support from friends and family, may help you stop problematic emotional eating habits.

Setting Realistic Goals

Setting realistic objectives is critical for staying motivated and monitoring progress after gastric bypass surgery. These objectives may be connected to weight reduction, physical fitness, eating habits, or other elements of health and well-being. It is critical to establish attainable objectives that are detailed, quantifiable, and time-constrained.

Breaking down big objectives into smaller, more manageable stages might help them seem more achievable and avoid overwhelm. Celebrating little accomplishments along the road might give the incentive to continue moving ahead. It's also important to be adaptable and open to change objectives as required depending on personal development and circumstances.

Embracing A New Lifestyle

Gastric bypass surgery requires a considerable lifestyle change, and adopting this new way of life is critical for long-term success. This involves developing healthy behaviors, creating a happy mentality, and prioritizing self-care. Surrounding yourself with a supporting network of friends, family, and healthcare experts may help you stay motivated and focused on your goals.

Learning to handle social settings, eating out, and holidays while following dietary requirements may need some adaptations, but it is fully possible with experience and forethought. Finding new ways to enjoy food, such as attempting new dishes or exploring various cuisines, may help make the post-surgery period more joyful and gratifying.

Finally, maintaining a healthy life after gastric bypass surgery means finding balance, listening to your body, and making decisions that promote your physical and mental well-being. You may optimize the advantages of surgery by combining healthy behaviors, practicing mindful eating, making realistic objectives, and adopting a new lifestyle.

Conclusion

Understanding gastric bypass surgery requires a comprehensive understanding of its advantages, hazards, and long-term consequences. This surgery has emerged as an important weapon in the fight against obesity and its related health issues, resulting in considerable weight reduction and improvement in a variety of comorbid conditions. However, it is critical to recognize the complexity and possible obstacles that accompany it.

For starters, gastric bypass surgery is a life-changing procedure for those who are very obese. It promotes weight reduction by modifying the structure of the digestive system and changing hormonal signals associated with appetite and fullness. This causes significant reductions in obesity-related illnesses such as type 2 diabetes, hypertension, and sleep apnea, eventually improving overall quality of life.

Furthermore, the long-term effectiveness of gastric bypass surgery is dependent on a strict commitment to lifestyle alterations such as dietary changes and frequent physical exercise. To get the best results and avoid weight return, patients must commit to a lifetime program of good eating and frequent exercise. Furthermore, regular medical monitoring and assistance from healthcare specialists are required to manage any nutritional shortages or issues that may develop after surgery.

However, gastric bypass surgery has dangers and restrictions. Infections, blood clots, and gastrointestinal leaks are all possible complications, underscoring the need to choose a skilled surgeon and do thorough preoperative examinations. Furthermore, patients may develop food intolerance, vitamin shortages, and psychosocial difficulties after surgery, demanding continuing assistance and counseling.

Furthermore, although gastric bypass surgery may result in considerable weight reduction and metabolic advantages, it is not a one-size-fits-all treatment. Patient selection parameters such as BMI, obesity-related health issues, and psychological preparation are critical in assessing eligibility for surgery. Individuals must also comprehend the procedure's irreversible nature and the possible influence on their lifestyle and food habits.

In conclusion, gastric bypass surgery is an effective weapon in the battle against obesity and its related health risks. It provides significant weight reduction and metabolic benefits, resulting in an improved quality of life for many people. However, it is critical to approach this choice with caution, assessing the rewards against the hazards and recognizing the lifetime commitment necessary for success. Patients may confidently traverse this transforming path and attain long-term health and well-being by receiving comprehensive information, support, and medical treatment.

THE END

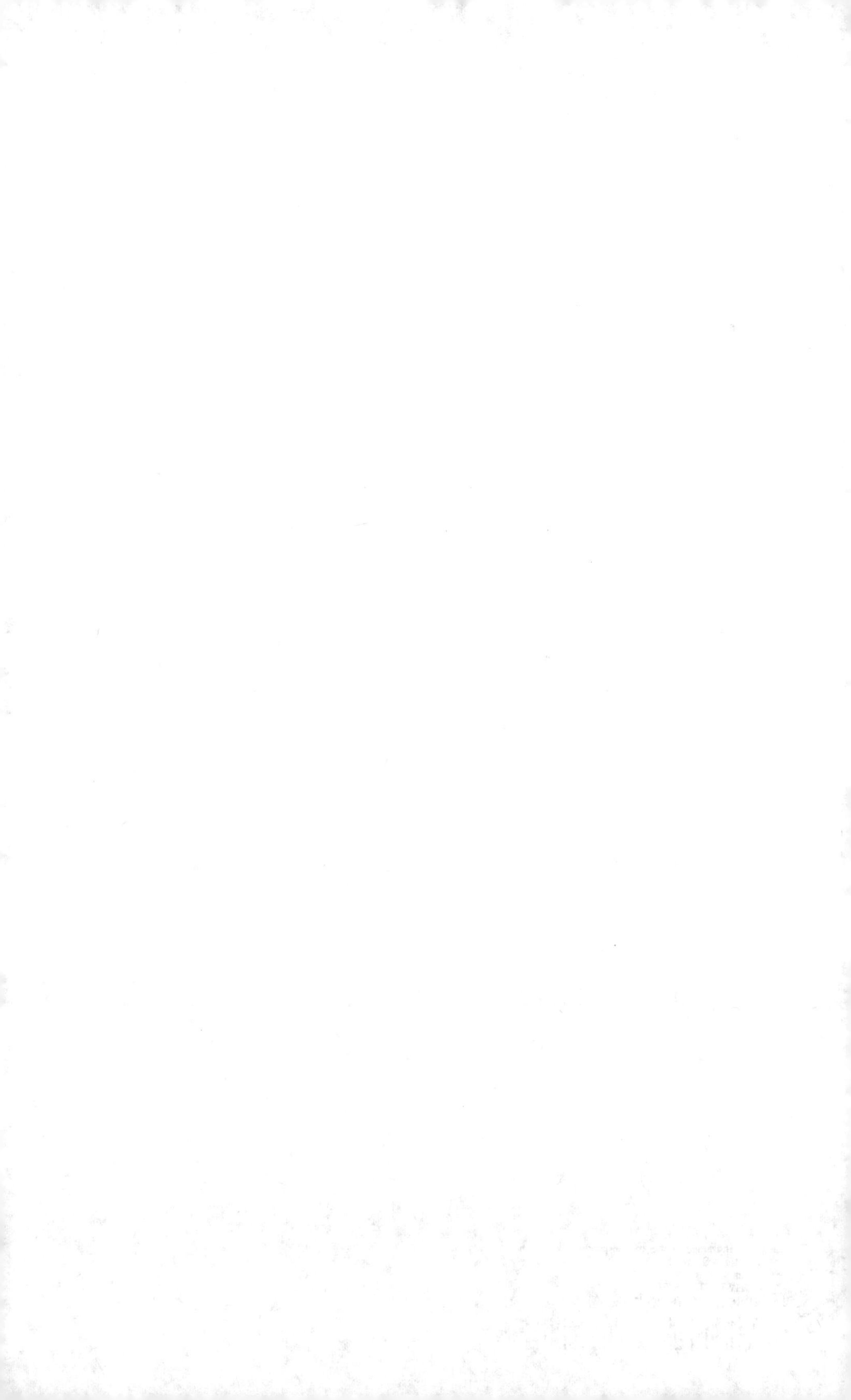

www.ingramcontent.com/pod-product-compliance
Lightning Source LLC
Chambersburg PA
CBHW061300250726
48653CB00002B/703